DIABETES
MEAL PREP

Table of Contents

DIABETES 1
    What is diabetes? 1
    What are the symptoms of diabetes? 1

MEAL PLANNING 2
    Diabetes meal plans made easy. 2
    Prep for quick meals. 2
    Make the right choices 2

HEALTHY FOOD CHOICES MADE EASY 3
    Eat right to feel good. 3
    Learn the keys to healthy eating. 3

DIABETES SUPERFOODS 4
    Diabetes Superfoods 4
        Beans 4
        Dark green leafy vegetables 4
        Citrus fruit 4
        Sweet potatoes 5
        Berries 5
        Tomatoes 5
        Fish high in omega-3 fatty acids 5
        Nuts 5
        Whole grains 5
        Milk and yogurt 6

FRUITS 7
    What are the best choices? 7
    Tips 7
        For carbohydrate counters 7
        For the plate method 7
        For using the glycemic index 8

Common fruits 8

HEALTHY-HEART 10

Choose the right fats—in moderation 10

Include those omega-3s 10

With less fat, sugar, and salt, more flavor 11

Trim the fat 11

UNDERSTANDING FOOD LABELS 12

Untangle packaging claims. 12

Put food labels to work 12

Making sense of food labels 12

Serving size 12

Amount per serving 13

Calories 13

Total carbohydrate 13

Get smart on carbs. 13

• Eat the most of these 14

• Eat some of these 14

• Try to eat less of these 14

Get to Know Carbs 14

Know the three types 15

RECIPE FOR DIABETIC PATIENTS 27

PEACH SMOOTHIE 27

Serves: 2 27

Ingredients: 27

Directions: 27

Comments: 27

ENGLISH MUFFIN BREAKFAST PIZZA 28

Serves: 1 28

Ingredients: 28

Directions: 28

Comments: 28

MULTI-BRAN MUFFINS 28

    Makes: 16 28

    Ingredients: 28

    Directions: 29

    Comments: 29

BREAKFAST SANDWICH 29

    Ingredients: 29

    Direction: 30

    Comments: 30

NORTHWEST BERRY PUFF 30

    Serves: 6 30

    Ingredients: 30

    Directions: 30

MUSHROOM OMELET 31

    Serves: 2 31

    Ingredients: 31

    Directions: 31

    Comments: 32

SAUSAGE STRATA 32

    Ingredients: 32

    Directions: 32

    Comments: 33

ROASTED TOMATILLO SALSA 33

    Ingredients: 33

    Direction: 33

EGGS TUDOR 33

    Ingredients: 33

    Directions: 34

    Comments: 34

SPINACH SALAD 34
    Ingredients: 34
    Directions: 35
    Comments: 35

KALE, LENTIL, & CHICKEN SALAD WITH MAPLE VINAIGRETTE 35
    Ingredients: 35
    Directions: 36
    Comments: 36

QUINOA SALAD WITH RICE & BLACK BEANS 36
    Serves: 6 36
    Ingredients: 36
    Directions: 37
    Comments: 37

ITALIAN SALAD 37
    Ingredients: 37
    Directions: 38

LENTILS, MINT & FETA FOR 2 38
    Serves: 2 38
    Ingredient: 38
    Directions: 38
    Comments: 39

ROASTED CAULIFLOWER, CHICKPEAS & OLIVES 39
    Serves: 6 39
    Ingredients: 39
    Directions: 40
    Comments: 40

GRILLED CHILES RELLENOS 40
    Ingredients: 40
    Directions: 40
    Comments: 41

BAKED LEEK & SWEET POTATO GRATIN 41
    Serves: 8 41
    Ingredients: 41
    Directions: 41
APPLE-GLAZED BABY CARROTS 42
    Ingredients: 42
    Directions: 42
ROASTED CARROTS WITH SHALLOTS & SAGE 42
    Serves: 2 42
    Ingredients: 42
    Directions: 43
    Comments: 43
MASHED CAULIFLOWER POTATOES 43
    Serves: 4 43
    Ingredients: 43
    Directions: 43
    Comments: 44
GARLIC MUSHROOMS 44
    Serves: 12 44
    Ingredients: 44
    Directions: 44
    Comments: 44
DECADENT BRUSSELS SPROUTS 44
    Serve: 4 44
    Ingredients: 44
    Directions: 45
    Comments: 45
SWEET POTATO SPEARS 45
    Serves: 4 45
    Ingredients: 45

- Directions 45
- **CURRIED LENTILS & CAULIFLOWER** 46
  - Ingredients: 46
  - Directions 46
- **CHICKEN & WHITE BEAN SOUP** 47
  - Ingredients: 47
  - Directions: 47
  - Comments: 47
- **TACO SOUP** 48
  - Serves: 4 48
  - Ingredients: 48
  - Directions: 48
  - Comments: 48
- **EGG, LEMON & RICE SOUP (AVGOLEMONO SOUPA)** 48
  - Serves: 8 48
  - Ingredients: 48
  - Directions: 49
  - Comments: 49
- **BEEF BARLEY SOUP** 49
  - Serves: 8 49
  - Ingredients: 49
  - Directions: 50
- **CHICKEN & VEGETABLE SOUP** 50
  - Serves: 4 50
  - Ingredients: 50
  - Directions: 50
  - Comments: 51
- **CURRY PUMPKIN SOUP** 51
  - Serves: 6 51
  - Ingredients: 51

- Directions: 51
  - Comments: 52
- TURKEY CHILI 52
  - Serves: 4 52
  - Ingredients: 52
  - Directions: 52
  - Comments: 52
- ITALIAN CHICKEN WITH CHICKPEAS 53
  - Serves: 4 53
  - Ingredients: 53
  - Directions: 53
  - Comments: 53
- CHICKEN TORTILLAS 53
  - Makes: 12 53
  - Ingredients: 53
  - Directions: 54
- SALSA TURKEY MEATLOAF 54
  - Serves: 6 54
  - Ingredients: 54
  - Directions: 54
- BARBEQUE PULLED CHICKEN 55
  - Serves: 8 55
  - Ingredients: 55
  - Directions: 55
- CILANTRO CITRUS CHICKEN 56
  - Serves: 4 56
  - Ingredients: 56
  - Directions: 56
- OVEN-FRIED CHICKEN 56
  - Serves: 4 56

Ingredients: 56

Directions: 57

Comments / Tips: 57

CHICKEN CASSOULET 57

Serves: 6 57

Ingredients: 57

Directions: 58

CHICKEN LO MEIN WITH PEANUT SAUCE 58

Serves: 6 (about 2 cups per serving) 58

Ingredients: 58

Directions: 59

Comment: 59

GRILLED FISH TACOS WITH CHIPOTLE-LIME DRESSING 60

Serves: 4 60

Ingredients: 60

Directions: 61

Comments: 61

APPLE-GLAZED SALMON 61

Serves: 2 61

Ingredients: 61

Directions: 62

POACHED WHITEFISH 62

Serves: 4 62

Ingredients: 62

Directions: 62

FARFALLE WITH SALMON, MINT, AND PEAS 63

Serves: 6 63

Ingredients: 63

Directions: 63

Comments: 63

GRILLED SALMON STEAKS WITH TARRAGON SAUCE 64
- Serves: 4 64
- Ingredients 64
- Directions: 64
- Comments: 64

DIABETES

What is diabetes?

The diabetic issue is a problem where the body does not process food as power appropriately. Most of the food we consume is developed into glucose or sugar to use our bodies' energy. The pancreas, a body near the stomach, makes an insulin hormone that helps glucose into our body cells. Either you can't get enough insulin in your body, or you can't do the same for your diabetes. It causes blood sugar to accumulate. It is why lots of people call diabetes mellitus" sugar." Diabetes may cause severe health complications, including cardiac disease, blindness, renal failure, and lower extremity amputations.

What are the symptoms of diabetes?

For diagnosis, people who think they might have diabetes need to visit a doctor. They may have the following symptoms, SOME or NONE:

- Sores that are slow to heal
- Dehydrated skin
- Excessive thirst
- Sudden vision changes
- Tingling or numbness in hands or feet
- Frequent urination
- Extreme hunger 1
- Feeling very tired much of the time
- Unexplained weight loss
- More infections than usual

Can diabetes be prevented?

The answer is yes;

A healthy meal can reduce and control the risk of developing diabetes.

MEAL PLANNING

Diabetes meal plans made easy.

No small challenge is timing meals to keep blood sugar levels controlled. To make your life simpler, look into these suggestions.

Prep for quick meals.

If you eat what you have on hand or stop on the closest road, or if your life is too busy, nutritious meals will make your seat more comfortable. Get tips on stocking up, so that fast, healthy meal ideas are always on hand.

Make the right choices

Meal prep is more than just what you are going to eat. What is healthy to treat diabetes is making the right decisions that work with your personal everyday life and preferences. Get the fundamentals down, and in no time, you will be a pro.

HEALTHY FOOD CHOICES MADE EASY

Eat right to feel good.

It's not essential to make healthy eating difficult. You can learn how to build an eating plan that's good for your body by following these essential tips.

Learn the keys to healthy eating.

It cannot be obvious to know what to consume. There's news on what is or isn't right for you wherever you turn. But the test of time has withstood a few essential tips. Here's what all healthy eating strategies have in common, regardless of what food you want. Included are:

- Less processed foods
- Less added sugar
- Fruits and vegetables
- Lean meats and plant-based sources of protein

DIABETES SUPERFOODS

Supercharge these ten foods full of vitamins, minerals, and fiber for your meal schedule.

Diabetes Superfoods

Superfood" is a word used mostly by food and beverage organizations to gain a food thought to have medical benefits; however, the Food and Drug Administration (FDA) does not have an official definition of the word." To ensure that there is scientific evidence to support the claims, the FDA controls the health claims permitted on food labels. The food list below is rich in vitamins, minerals, antioxidants, and fiber, beneficial for general health and help prevent illnesses.

Beans

Renal, pinto, navy, or black beans are packaged with vitamins and minerals such as magnesium and potassium. They're still very high in fiber.

Beans may have carbohydrates, but 1/2 cup still contains as much protein as an ounce of beef without the saturated fat. It would help if you used canned beans to save time; make sure that you drain and clean them and get away from the salt as best as you can.

Dark green leafy vegetables

The dark green leafy vegetables, packed with vitamins and minerals such as vitamins A, C, E, and K, iron, calcium, and potassium, are spinach, collards, and kale. The calories and carbohydrates of these powerhouse foods are also low. For salads, soups, and stews, try adding dark leafy vegetables.

Citrus fruit

Grapefruits, oranges, lemons, and limes, or select your favorites to get part of your day-to-day dosage of fiber, vitamin C, folate, and potassium.

Sweet potatoes

A starchy vegetable filled with fiber and vitamin A isis also a decent potassium and vitamin C source.

Are you craving a sweet thing? Instead of a regular potato, try the sweet potato and sprinkle cinnamon on top.

Berries

What if your favorites are blueberries, strawberries, or a different variety? Nonetheless, they are all made of antioxidants, vitamins, and fiber. Berries can be a perfect way to fulfill your sweet tooth, and vitamin C, vitamin K, manganese, potassium, and fiber offer a bonus.

Tomatoes

The good news is that you eat essential nutrients such as vitamin C, vitamin E, and potassium, regardless of how you like your tomatoes, pureed, raw, or in a sauce.

Fish high in omega-3 fatty acids

Omega-3 fats can help reduce the risk of inflammation and heart disease. Often, fish rich in these healthy fats are referred to as "fatty fish." In this category, salmon is well known. Other fatty omega-3 fish include herring, sardines, mackerel, salmon, and albacore tuna. To avoid the sugars and extra calories in breaded and fried fish, choose fish broiled, baked, or grilled.

Nuts

In having primary healthy fats and helping to control hunger, an ounce of nuts will go a long way. They sell magnesium and fiber also. Few nuts and grains, such as nuts and linseed, are healthy omega-3 fatty acids.

Whole grains

It's all the grain you're after. The first ingredient on the packaging should include the word "whole." Whole grains are rich in vitamins and minerals such as magnesium, B vitamins, chromium, iron, and folate. They're still a decent source of fiber. Such examples of whole grains are whole oats, quinoa, whole-grain barley, and farrow.

Milk and yogurt

You may have learned that milk and yogurt will help develop healthy bones and teeth. Besides calcium, many milk and yogurt products are fortified to make them a good source of vitamin D. Further evidence is emerging on the association between vitamin D and good health. Milk and yogurt contain carbs that can be a factor in your food preparation when you have diabetes. Look for yogurt items with reduced fat content and added sugar.

FRUITS

Fruit contains starch, but you ought to include that as part of your meal schedule. Eating a piece of fresh fruit or fruit salad for dessert is a perfect way to please your sweet tooth and get the extra calories you're looking for.

What are the best choices?

The better fruit options are those that are fresh, frozen, or canned without added sugars.

- Watch for terms like "packed in its juices," "unsweetened," or no added sugar." when selecting canned fruit.
- Dried fruit and 100% fruit juice are both nutritious options, but serving sizes are limited enough that they might not be as full as other choices.

Tips

For carbohydrate counters

A small piece of whole fruit or roughly 1/2 cup of frozen or canned fruit has about 15 grams of carbohydrate. Servings with most new berries and melons are 3/4 to 1 cup. Fruit juice will range from 1/3 to 1/2 cup for 15 grams of carbohydrate.

Just two tablespoons of dried fruit such as raisins or dried cherries produce 15 grams of carbohydrate, so be alert about your portion sizes!

Fruit should be consumed in return for other carbohydrates in your meal schedule, such as starches, wheat, or milk.

For the plate method

If you use a plating process, including a small piece of whole fruit or a 1/2 cup of fruit salad for dessert is a perfect complement to the non-starchy vegetables, a small amount of starch and protein food on your plate.

For using the glycemic index

Many fruits have a low glycemic index (GI) due to their fructose and fiber content. Pineapples and melons have medium GI values, as do some dried fruit such as dates, raisins, and sweetened cranberries.

Overall, the fruit is promoted by using the glycemic index to guide food choices—so enjoy.

Common fruits

A list of common fruits is set out below:

- Apples
- Apricots
- Avocado
- Banana
- Blackberries
- Blueberries
- Cantaloupe
- Cherries
- Dried fruit such as:
    - Cherries
    - Cranberries
    - Dates
    - Figs
    - Prunes
    - Raisins
- Grapefruit
- Grapes
- Honeydew melon
- Kiwi
- Mango
- Nectarine
- Orange

- Papaya
- Peaches
- Pears
- Pineapple
- Plums
- Raspberries
- Strawberries
- Tangerines
- Watermelon

HEALTHY-HEART

Only minor cooking improvements can help reduce the risk of heart disease. Your heart and blood vessels will be secured by:

- Make options for foods that contain healthier fats and reducing those containing fewer healthy fats.
- Moving to a good weight and keeping it, it's hard work but worth it.
- A decrease in foods that are high in sodium will make a difference, particularly if you have high blood pressure.

Choose the right fats—in moderation

Foods such as frozen chips, cookies, baked goods, fried foods, red meat, and cooked meats such as bacon and sausage are rich in saturated fats that increase the bad cholesterol.

New vegetables, whole grains, and berries are low in fat and rich in vitamins, minerals, and dietary fibers that can reduce heart disease risk. Good fats supply you with almonds, avocados, and plant-based oils (such as olive, peanut, and safflower oils, to name a few). When frying, pay attention to the number of oils and butter you apply to reduce the net calories to assist in weight loss. Butter is rich in saturated fat, so try to reduce the volume you're using.

Include those omega-3s

Foods rich in omega-3 fats are beneficial for the wellbeing of your heart, including "fatty" fish such as salmon, albacore tuna, herring, rainbow trout, mackerel, and sardines.

Soya bean products, walnuts, flaxseed, and canola oil are other foods that contain omega-3 fatty acids. Aim to do this daily in your eating schedule, but pay care to your servings since a little quantity goes a long way.

With less fat, sugar, and salt, more flavor

Instead of salt, butter, lard, or other harmful fats, consider using herbs and spices for taste. To add flavor to your rice, here are a couple of ideas:

- On steamed tomatoes, broiled salmon, potatoes, salads, or pasta, squeeze fresh lemon juice or lime juice.
- Try herbs and spices that are salt-free. A perfect alternative is new herbs, too.
- Without the weak stuff, onion and garlic add lots of flavors.
- Try marinades for meat with good oils, herbs, and spices dependent on vegetables.

Trim the fat

Cut out the apparent fat from poultry and beef. To make the fat drip off, roast food on a rack. Choose lean meat cuts and strip the skin off poultry until you consume it.

UNDERSTANDING FOOD LABELS

Untangle packaging claims.

You're not alone if you get stumbled upon nutritional quality statements. Fat-free vs. fat low vs. fat limited. Cholesterol-low vs. cholesterol-lowered. It's complicated because when you try to make the best decisions, it can be difficult.

Put food labels to work

The labels on foods from Nutrition Information are the secret to making the right decisions. From knowing serving sizes and quantity per serving to carbs, fat, and more, we'll cover the basics so that these marks make shopping easy for you.

Making sense of food labels

It is not easy to try and figure out nutritional data on labels and packaging. The good news is we're here to help. If you use carb counting to prepare your meals, these product labels are handy!

If you get stumbled upon claims of food quality, you're not alone. Fat-free vs. low fat vs. diminished fat. Cholesterol-low vs. cholesterol-lowered. It's complicated, and when you want to make the right decisions, it can be cruel.

Serving size

Begin by looking at the scale of the serve. The serving size specified is the basis for all the details on the box. That means that if you consume more, you get more calories, carbohydrates, etc., than what is mentioned.

Amount per serving

The details on the package's left side indicate the total amount of different nutrients in a single food serving. To equate the labeling of related foods, use these figures.

Calories

Think of them as the energy the body absorbs and uses for body activities. Calories are a unit of energy. How many calories do you need? Are you worried? Conversation with a certified nutritionist for dietitians (RD/RDN).

Total carbohydrate

The complete carbohydrate mark contains all three forms of carbohydrate: sugar, starch, and fiber. It is essential to use total grams when measuring carbs or to select which foods to include. Below the overall carbohydrate (carbs), you can describe the forms of carbohydrates throughout your diet.

Get smart on carbs.

When you consume or drink foods containing carbohydrates—also known as carbs—the body breaks certain carbs down into glucose (a form of sugar) and increases the amount of glucose throughout your blood. Your body uses glucose for food to keep you running all day. It is what you probably know as "blood glucose" or "blood sugar." When it comes to diabetes treatment, the carbohydrates you eat contribute an essential part. When the body splits the carbohydrates into glucose, the pancreas releases insulin to help your cells digest the glucose.

If someone's blood glucose—or blood sugar—is too high, it's called hyperglycemia. There are a few reasons for 'highs,' including not having enough insulin in your bloodstream to absorb glucose in your blood or cells in your body that do not respond efficiently to the insulin released, leaving excess glucose in your blood. Low blood glucose is considered to be hypoglycemia. "Lows" can also be caused by not eating enough carbohydrates or by a drug deficiency. In short, the carbohydrates we eat affect our blood sugar—so balancing is essential!

There are three significant types of carbohydrates in food: starch, sugar, and fiber. You can find on the nutrition labels for the products you purchase, the word "total carbohydrate" applies to all three of these forms. The goal is to use nutrient-dense carbs, which ensures high fiber, vitamins and minerals, and low in added sugars, sodium, and unsanitary fats. When selecting foods containing carbohydrates:

- **Eat the most of these**

Raw, unprocessed, non-starchy vegetables. Non-starchy foods such as spinach, cucumbers, broccoli, tomatoes, and green beans contain a lot of fiber and a relatively small amount of carbohydrate, which has a lower effect on blood sugar. Remember, these should make up half of your plate according to the Plate Process!

- **Eat some of these**

Whole, minimally processed carbohydrate items. They are the starchy carbs that contain fruit such as tomatoes, blueberries, strawberries, and cantaloupe. Entire grains such as brown rice, full wheat bread, whole grain pasta, and oatmeal; starchy vegetables such as corn, green peas, sweet potatoes, pumpkins, plantains; and beans and as black beans, kidney beans, chickpeas, and green lentils. If you are using the Plate Process, the food in this segment can make up about a quarter of your plate.

- **Try to eat less of these**

Refined, heavily processed starch and sugar-added items. They include sugary beverages such as soda, sweet tea, juice, processed grains such as white bread, white rice, sugary cereal, and desserts and snacks such as cakes, biscuits, candy, and chips.

Get to Know Carbs

Carbohydrates or "carbs" are getting a lot of attention these days, and it's no secret that carbs will influence blood sugars (blood glucose). You may wonder if you're going to eat less of them or even eat them at all. You aren't alone!

Carbs come in several different ways, but the three primary ones are starch, sugar, and fiber. When consuming processed goods, the word "total carbohydrate" refers to all three types of food. So how much is the right amount of money?

Let's begin with the fundamentals of it. All food is comprised of three essential nutrients: starch, protein, and fat. All three of you need to stay safe, but each person wants a different amount when selecting carbs; the trick to choosing complex carbs—the ones that give you the best of your bucks in terms of vitamins, minerals, and fiber.

Refined foods tend to be high in carbs, mainly processed carbohydrates, which are more likely to cause your blood sugar to rise, while still being very low in vitamins, minerals, and fiber—giving carbs a bad rap. Yet choosing fewer refined carb meals and paying attention to how much you consume will make a significant difference in your blood sugar and general health.

Now let's dive through the kinds of foods with carbohydrates and how to pick nutrient-dense foods.

Know the three types

There are three primary types of carbohydrates in food: starches, sugars, and fiber. Starch—or complex carbohydrates—includes starchy vegetables, dried beans, and grains. Sugars include those naturally occurring (like fruit) and added (like cookies). And fiber comes from vegetable food vs. animal products, such as eggs, beef, or fish.

Starch
Try targeting whole, minimally processed carbohydrate foods. If you are using the Plate Process, the food in this segment can make up about a quarter of your plate. Foods rich in starch contain:

- Starchy vegetables such as corn, winter squash, and potatoes
- Legumes and pulses, including lentils, beans (such as kidney beans, pinto beans, and black beans and peas (think split peas and black-eyed peas)
- Carbohydrates, including wheat foods such as pasta, bread, crackers, peas, barley, rice, etc.
- Whole grains are simply that, the whole plant that was grown and dried with no refining. They offer fiber and essential vitamins, including B and E, and other minerals required for optimum health.

Asking what the deal is with the 'refined grained,' these foods have nearly been refined. All the valuable fibers, vitamins, and minerals ordinarily absent from the whole grains are removed from external layers and more nutrient pieces of the crop. There are regulations in force that guarantee that necessary vitamins and minerals are added back in after manufacturing to prevent diseases caused by vitamin and mineral deficiency, which is what "enriched" means when you see it on the bottle. Bottom line: when reading the list of ingredients, look for items that list "whole grain" or whole wheat" as the first ingredient rather than "enriched."

Sugar

Sugar is a different type of carbohydrate. There are two major categories here:

- All-natural sugars such as those in milk or fruit
- Additional sugars that are added during manufacturing, such as daily soda, desserts, and baked goods;

You may have encountered added sugars alluded to by other names—or you may have seen one of them on the product label. Dextrose, fructose, lactose, table sugar, beet sugar, butter, corn syrup, turbinado, and agave are only a handful of various added sugars.

Sugar Substitutes

Sugar replacements, high-intensity sweeteners, chemical sweeteners, non-nutritive sweeteners, low-calorie sweeteners – with so many new items on the market, it's easy to understand how the consumer would have a hard time keeping up with evolving patterns. Luckily, we're here to help you break it down.

First of all, the U.S. The Food and Drug Administration (FDA) has reviewed a range of drugs and has licensed or accepted them as healthy for the public, particularly people with diabetes. There are the following:

- Advantame
- Saccharin
- Neotame
- AcesulfameK
- Luo Han Guo (or monk fruit)
- Sucralose
- Aspartame

- Stevia

The liver does not break these items down, but they move through our system without supplying calories. For certain people, the use of these products is an excellent alternative to sugar. Improved long-term blood sugar, weight, and cardiometabolic health (think: heart and metabolism) may benefit from a possible reduction in calories and carbohydrates.

The sweeteners themselves do not add calories, although certain foods that use these additives may include calories from other ingredients and carbohydrates. A word of warning: Claims such as "sugar-free," "reduced sugar," or no sugar added" are not inherently carbohydrate-free or less carbohydrate-free than the initial food edition. For this reason, we propose that you read the label for nutrition information and understand how many carbohydrates and calories you consume.

It may sound like music to some people's ears, but the benefits are not always as a straight cut. No calories, no carbohydrates. There is no strong indication that sugar substitutes improve long-term blood sugar, weight, or cardiometabolic fitness.

Using sugar alternatives, therefore, would not produce an unnatural, healthier alternative. It only means that it's less unhealthy.

Bottom line
- For certain people, sugar replacements are great alternatives to sugar, but not a seamless match for everybody. It is a personal preference.
- If you're attempting to decrease your sugar or sugar replacement intake, proceed slowly. E.g., begin by substituting water or a no-calorie drink for one soda or juice.
- A perfect alternative will always be water! If you start to find yourself getting bored with only drink, fruits or herbs like this sparkling strawberry mint-flavored water will still spruce it up.

Sugar alcohols
Sugar alcohol is a substitute for sugar that has fewer calories per gram than sugars and starches. Examples of sugar alcohol are sorbitol, xylitol, and mannitol. If a product produces alcohol from sugar, it will be classified under Total Carbohydrate on the bottle. It is important to note that sugar-alcoholic products are not necessarily low in carbohydrates or calories. And only because on the outside a box says "sugar-free" does not

mean that it is free of calories or carbohydrates. Still, check the grams of total carbohydrate and calories on the bottle.

What are Sugar Alcohols?

The bulk of replacements for sugar taste much sweeter than sugar. Since they are so sweet, only a small amount of sugar with almost no calories must have the same sweetness.

Sugar alcohols are less sweet than sugar, unlike other "high intensity" sweeteners, but they contain fewer calories per gram, making them a "low-calorie" sweetener.

Don't let you get misled by the term "alcohol," sugar alcohols aren't the same as the alcohol that allows you to get a buzz." In this situation, the word "alcohol" is concerned about the structure of the molecule, so don't worry, it's just a chemical issue.

How Are Sugar Alcohols Used?

In-home cooking or in packets at the coffee bar, sugar alcohols are not typically used, although they can be used in certain "sugar-free" foods, including chewing gum, sweets, ice cream, and fruit spreads. They are also widely used in toothpaste, mouthwash, and cough drops as a sweetener.

"The ingredients may also contain sugar alcohols in products labeled as "diet," "sugar-free," or no sugar added. If a food contains sugar alcohols, you can find "Sugar Alcohol" listed under Total Carbohydrates on the Nutrition Facts label. You should then check the list of ingredients to see which alcohols have been added to the sugar.

"Xylitol, erythritol, sorbitol, and maltitol are typical sugar alcohols that you can notice (they usually end in the letters-ol, as does "alcohol" sugar, which may be helpful to locate them in the ingredient list quickly).

Do Sugar Alcohols Raise Blood Sugar?

Sugar Alcohols are carbohydrates that can increase blood sugar. Sugar-free" foods containing sugar alcohols are not carbohydrate- or calorie-free, as you will notice in the Nutrition Facts label to the right!"

Sugar alcohols, however, are absorbed differently from other carbohydrates by the body, and some may raise the blood sugar by a little while others may not increase it at all.

Erythritol, for instance, is a form of alcohol that does not increase blood sugar. It has been widespread in low-carb "keto" foods as an ingredient for this cause. Erythritol can also be sold in some supermarkets and can be used for home cooking, but you can even see it as an ingredient in low-carb cake recipes.

What Might Sugar Alcohols Do in Other Parts of The Body?

Sugar alcohols, unlike regular sugar, do not promote cavities. Xylitol, a form of sugar alcohol used in sugar-free chewing gum, may help avoid cavities.

Many sugar alcohols, especially when ingested in large quantities, can cause gas, bloating, and stomach aches and specific individuals may be more susceptible than others to this effect.

When eating 'sugar-free' or other foods sweetened with sugar alcohol, if you have an irritated stomach, read the ingredients and see what kind of sugar alcohol is in the drink. You will choose to stop or cut down on how much you consume in one sitting, foods that contain that sort of sugar alcohol.

Bottom line

Alcohols from sugar are safe to eat and can be a healthy choice for people with diabetes. However, when consumed in significant doses, they can cause digestive problems, and some sugar alcohols can increase blood sugar.

"Sugar-free" does not mean free from sugars! To see the sugar-free foods' carbohydrate content, read the mark.

As long as you count the carbs, sugar-free meals will work into your diet schedule. To see how the blood sugar changes, monitor blood sugar 1 1/2- 2 hours after consuming a sugar alcohol meal.

As usual, the dietitian or diabetes health care staff will help you determine if the right alternative is to use some form of sugar alternatives in your food schedule.

Fiber

Fiber comes from foods dependent on plants, including bananas, vegetables, and intact whole grains. Fiber behaves like the actual scrub brush of your body, which travels through your digestive system, bringing many unpleasant things along with it. It leaves us feeling full, too, and helps lower cholesterol. Consuming higher-fiber foods will also boost your metabolism, help you control your blood pressure, and reduce your heart disease risk. These are not the only advantages.

It is recommended that people with diabetes and those at risk of diabetes consume at least the same amount of dietary fiber recommended by all Americans. The Dietary Recommendations for Americans require a minimum of 14 grams of fiber per 1,000 calories, with at least half the grains being whole-intact. In the Dietary Guidelines for Americans (DGA), you can find unique recommendations for your age group and gender.

Bear in mind that if you haven't eaten many high-fiber foods regularly, slowly increasing your consumption is significant. And when they are safe for you, it will take time for the body to adapt. Gas, bloating, or constipation may be caused by a sudden rise in eating foods high in fiber (especially foods with added fiber or using supplements). As fiber needs water to pass around your body, make sure you drink enough water too!

Good sources of dietary fiber include:
Beans and vegetables (think navy beans, little white beans, split peas, chickpeas, lentils, pinto beans), and pulses (like lentils and peas),

Fruit and vegetables, particularly with edible skin like pears, apples and beans and edible seeds (like berries) Fruit and vegetables

Try various types of nuts (pumpkin seeds, almonds, sunflower seeds, pistachios, peanuts are a decent source of fiber and healthy fat, but monitor portion sizes since they often have a limited number of calories!)

Whole grains such as:

Quinoa, barley, farro, and brown rice

Whole pasta with wheat

Whole-grain cereal products, including whole wheat, wheat bran, and oats

The food that is natural in fiber contains at a minimum of two and a half grams, is primarily regarded as a good source," while the food called "excellent source" provides over five grams of fiber per serving.

While it is better to receive fiber from your diets, chat about whether fiber substitution can be offered to your diabetes care team.

Fats

Full fat shows you how much fat a piece of food contains. Consider replacing food with foods rich in monounsaturated or polyunsaturated fats. To decrease the chances of heart disease, they are rich in saturated fat or trans fat.

Fats

Carbohydrates, usually referred to as carbs, attract all the publicity in the treatment of diabetes, no doubt about it. However, as part of a healthy diet, another essential nutrient to remember is fat. And if it seems counter-intuitive to what you would think, our bodies play a crucial role in eating the right amount of the right kind of fat.

Fat cushions tissues retain energy, insulate the body from components, stimulate cell growth, and more. The trick is to look after the fat bits, so the fat is better per gram of calories. To minimize the risk of type 2 diabetes, cardiovascular disease, certain cancers, and other health issues, consuming the correct fat types is also significant.

Four significant fat forms are available: saturated, trans, monounsaturated, and polyunsaturated fat. The U.S. Diabetes Association advises that more single- and polyunsaturated fats be used in your diet than saturation and trans fats. The Nutrition Facts mark on food items lists specific categories of fat.

It's important to remember what we mean when we say cholesterol when we talk about fat. There are two types: the kind present in our blood, known as cholesterol in the blood, and the cholesterol that we consume, known as cholesterol throughout the diet.

In the body, blood cholesterol plays an essential role and is the starting point for hormones, cell structures, vitamin D, and more to be formed. For these applications, the body contains more than enough cholesterol, but it can still absorb tiny quantities from the foods you consume.

You are at higher risk of heart failure because the average cholesterol in the blood is too high. However, dietary cholesterol has less effect on this figure than generally thought, contrary to common opinion. Increased blood cholesterol for many people plays a much more critical role in saturated and trans fat, leading to increased heart disease risk. Since saturated fat is often high in foods that are usually high in dietary cholesterol, it is most comfortable to concentrate on limiting saturated fat.

Speak to a certified nutritionist (RD/RDN) or a health care professional to find out what priorities are right for you.

Monounsaturated fat

Monounsaturated fats are a part of a balanced, nutritional diet due to our cores' healing properties. Our low-density lipoprotein (LDL) cholesterol, an important marker for heart health, has been shown to decrease these fats. There is no need for monounsaturated fats to be listed on the Nutrition Facts bottle, but they are mostly for foods where they are a good source.

The monounsaturated fat sources include:

- Peanut butter and peanut oil
- Safflower Oil
- Avocado
- Canola oil
- Olive oil (look for low/reduced sodium) and olives
- Nuts like almonds, cashews, pecans, and peanuts

Consider substituting olive or canola oil instead of butter, margarine, or shortening while frying to have more monounsaturated fats in your diet. A simple way to consume more single-unsaturated fats is to sprinkle a few nuts on a sandwich, yogurt, or cereal. But make sure to be mindful of the servings you consume. These items are rich in calories, like all fats.

Polyunsaturated fat

As part of a healthy, nutritious diet, polyunsaturated fats are another essential fat to use. This fat reduces LDL cholesterol and the chances for heart disease and stroke, just as monounsaturated fat.

Two types of polyunsaturated fat are Omega-3 and Omega-6 fatty acids, both associated with better heart health. These fats must be included as part of a balanced diet as they are considered essential fatty acids, and our body cannot manufacture them.

Omega 3s origins include:

- Canola Oil
- Flaxseeds and flaxseed oil
- Walnuts
- Chia seeds
- Oily fish (salmon, sardines, herring, mackerel, tuna)

Sources of Omega 6s include:

- Canola oil
- Walnuts
- Tofu
- Flaxseed and flaxseed oil
- Eggs
- Sunflower seeds
- Peanut butter

Saturated fat

It kind of fat will increase your cholesterol and, consequently, your risk of developing heart disease. It is one of the fats in our diet that should be reduced. Usually, in animal products and tropical oils, reliable at room temperature, this fat is contained.

Items of animal origin containing saturated fat include:

- Lard
- Poultry skin (example: chicken, turkey, etc.)
- Fatback and salt pork
- Gravy made with meat drippings
- High-fat meats such as standard ground beef, bologna, ham, bacon, spareribs, and hot dogs
- Butter
- Cream sauces
- High-fat milk products, such as full-fat cheese, yogurt, whole milk, ice cream, 2% oil, and sour cream.

Saturated fat-containing oils include:

- Coconut and coconut oil
- Palm oil and palm kernel oil

Grams of saturated fat are classified under "total fat" on the Nutrition Facts label. The goal is to get saturated fat from less than 10 percent of one's calories. Someone eating a 2,000-calorie diet, for instance, should strive for saturated fat of 20 grams or less. Speak to the nutritionist to find out the right goal for you.

Trans fat

Trans fats are formed by a process called hydrogenation when liquid oil is turned into solid fat. Trans fat can be detrimental to blood cholesterol levels, much as saturated fat. It is more dangerous than saturated fat, and by eliminating foods containing it, you want to eat as less trans fat as possible for a heart-healthy diet.

On the Nutrition Facts mark, trans fats are identified, making it easy to recognize certain foods. Bear in mind, however, that if a food does not contain at least 0.5 grams or more of trans fat, the label will say 0 grams. You should read the ingredients list on food labels to remove as much trans fat as possible. Look for terms such as hydrogenated or partly hydrogenated crude. Avoid foods that come first on the ingredients list where liquid oil is listed.

Among the origins of trans fat are:

- Processed food with hydrogenated oil or partly hydrogenated oil, such as snacks (crackers and chips) and baked goods (muffins, cookies, and cakes)
- Margarine
- Shortening
- Some things for fast food, such as french fries

Sodium

The chemical name for salt is sodium. Blood sugar does not affect it. However, the risk of elevated blood pressure and heart failure is raised by excess dietary sodium. You may taste how spicy they are, such as pickles or pork, for some meats. But in certain foods, including salad dressings, lunch meat, canned soups, and other processed foods, there is still secret salt. Reading labels will help you identify these unknown origins and compare the salt of various foods. If you have diabetes or not, the general prescription is 2300 milligrams (mg) or less a day. Speak with the health care team to figure out the right goal to have elevated blood pressure.

Please speak to a licensed nutritionist (RD/RDN) or a health care professional to find out better what plans are right for you when it comes to fats.

"Net carbs" and other nutrient claims

Calories Claims
- Free of calories: less than five calories per serving
- Low-calorie: 40 or fewer calories per serving

Requests for total, saturated and trans fat
- Calorie-free: less than 0.5 grams of fat
- Free saturated fat: less than 0.5 grams of saturated fat
- Free trans fat: less than 0.5 grams of trans fat
- Low weight: 3 or fewer grams of total fat
- Low saturated fat: 1 gram or less of saturated fat
- Reduced-fat or lower fat: at least 25% less fat than the standard version

Claims for sodium
- Free of sodium or salt: less than 5 mg of sodium per serving
- Quite a little sodium: 35 mg or less of sodium
- Small sodium: 140 mg sodium or less
- Less sodium or decreased sodium: at least 25 percent less sodium than the regular version

Cholesterol Claims
- Independence from cholesterol: less than 2 mg per serving
- Low cholesterol: 20 mg or smaller
- Less cholesterol or reduced cholesterol: at least 25 percent fewer cholesterol than the standard version

Claims for sugar
- Sugar-free: less than 0.5 grams of sugar per serving
- Reduced sugar: a minimum of 25% less sugar per serving than the standard edition
- Little added sugar or no added sugar: no added sugar or ingredient containing sugar is added during the production of Fiber Claims

Fiber Claims
- Good fiber: per serving, 5 grams of fiber or more
- Effective fiber source: 2.5 to 4.9 grams of fiber per serving.

RECIPE FOR DIABETIC PATIENTS

PEACH SMOOTHIE

Serves: 2

Ingredients:
- One medium fresh, peeled, pitted, and chopped peach
- ½ c skim milk 14 oz non-fat vanilla yogurt
- One c ice cubes ground cinnamon, to taste

Directions:
1. In a blender, put the peach, milk, yogurt, and ice together. Blend until perfectly smooth. Turn the pump off to scrape the blender side with a rubber spatula. Again, blend.
2. Pour two glasses of the mixture and sprinkle each one with a little cinnamon. For once, serve. (If you want to be fancy, you should garnish it with strawberries.)

Comments:
A refreshing, easy breakfast drink or an afternoon snack

You should replace your beloved frozen fruit if the fresh fruit is not in season. Pick a product that does not have sugar added.

ENGLISH MUFFIN BREAKFAST PIZZA

Serves: 1

Ingredients:

- Two Tbs of reduced cream cheese fat
- One tsp of fat-reduced sour cream
- 1/2 English Muffins
- One thin, peeled, and sliced ripe peach
- 1/2 tsp of soft brown cinnamon ground sugar, to taste.

Directions:

1. Preheat the broiler.
2. Combine the cream cheese and the sour cream in a little tub.
3. Spread uniformly over half of the English muffin.
4. Arrange the roof of peach slices. Using cinnamon and brown sugar to scatter.
5. Broil for about 2 minutes before the cheese browns around the edges.
6. Halve or break into quarters and eat soft.

Comments:

For the best' bang for the buck', pick a whole grain, high-fiber English muffin.

MULTI-BRAN MUFFINS

Makes: 16

Ingredients:

- One and a half c oat bran
- One Tbs baking powder
- One c wheat bran

- One tsp baking soda ¼ c orange juice
- One c Splenda brown sugar blend
- One c low-fat milk
- One Tbs cinnamon half c canola oil
- One tsp orange peel
- One c egg substitute
- One c raisins or craisins
- One c flour
- One c walnuts, chopped
- Half c whole wheat flour
- Half c cinnamon chips, optional.

Directions:

1. Spray with cooking spray on muffin cups or line with muffin sheets—Preheat the oven to 375 degrees F.
2. In a big tub, add six ingredients (egg substitution oat bran); sit 5 minutes.
3. In another cup, combine the next seven dried ingredients (through the orange peel). Add to the mixture of bran and stir only before mixed.
4. If used, add raisins/craisins, nuts, and chips. Scoop and bake in muffin cups for 18 minutes. 5. Let cool for 5 minutes in the pan, then remove the muffins and cool completely.

Comments:

In plastic sandwich bags, it will freeze. Remove the muffins from the bag and place them on a plate if you want to eat them. To defrost, microwave for 20 seconds, switch the pan, and microwave for 15 more seconds.

BREAKFAST SANDWICH

Ingredients:

- One whole-grain muffin of England break and toasted (in the frozen food section, I use Food for Life sprouted muffins)

- One frozen pre-cooked sausage patty, heated to the mustard in a microwave,

Direction:

1. Dissolve a little mustard toasted muffin, add a sandwich, and eat the sausage.

Comments:

It's swift, not spiking up my blood sugar. Practical, fast food concepts facilitate life!

NORTHWEST BERRY PUFF

Serves: 6

Ingredients:

- Two large eggs
- One large egg white
- Half c fat-free milk
- Half c all-purpose flour
- One Tbs sugar pinch salt
- Two c fresh berries of your choice
- One Tbs powdered sugar cooking spray

Directions:

1. Heat the furnace to 400°F. Use cooking spray to spray a 10-inch glass pie pan or oven-safe skillet.
2. In a medium dish, beat the eggs and egg whites. Whisk the milk in it. Whisk in the rice, sugar, and salt gently. Please place them in a prepared pan and cook for 15 minutes. Reduce the heat to 350 degrees F and bake for 10 minutes or until the batter is browned and puffed.

3. Remove and slip from the oven onto the serving tray. Cover with the fruit (slice into bite-sized pieces if strawberries are used and sprinkle with powdered sugar. Break and serve into six wedges.

MUSHROOM OMELET

Serves: 2

Ingredients:
- Six oz fresh mushrooms, such as shitake, portobello, or button
- Two scallions, white parts only, thinly sliced
- ¼ tsp minced thyme
- ¼ tsp minced basil
- One Tbs chopped fresh flat-leaf parsley freshly ground pepper Eight oz liquid egg substitute
- Two sprigs fresh parsley, for garnish cooking spray

Directions:
1. Using cooking spray to spray a small non-stick skillet and heat over high heat for 1 minute.
2. Attach the mushrooms and the scallions and cook over high heat until the mushrooms are cooked through.
3. In a shallow cup, extract and apply the herbs and seasonings.
4. Spray the same cooking spray on the pan and use part of the egg replacement. Cook over medium heat to allow the uncooked eggs to flow down, raising the eggs' sides.
5. Flip the omelet gently to brown the other side until the omelet has been lightly browned.
6. Spoon the omelet with half the mushroom mixture and fold in half. Switch to a plate and remain cozy, sealed with foil, in a warm oven.
7. Repeat; a second omelet is made. On each omelet, put a sprig of parsley.

Comments:

For or in addition to the mushrooms, substitute some vegetables. Sautéing red and orange baby peppers are one of our favorites. They bring lovely colors and taste fantastic.

SAUSAGE STRATA

Ingredients:

- ¾ c shredded low- fat
- Two c 1% milk cheddar cheese
- One lb chicken or turkey sausage
- Eight slices, good quality
- One and a Half c egg substitute white bread, crusts cooking spray removed and cut into cubes
- One and a Half c roasted tomatillo salsa (recipe follows)

Directions:

1. Remove the sausage wrapper and discard it. Crumble and brown in a non-stick pan, stirring and splitting with a wooden spoon. Move to a paper-towel-lined plate with a slotted spoon.
2. In a large tub, mix milk and egg replacement.
3. Coat a baking dish of 9 "x9" with cooking oil. Place aside 1/4 cup of sliced cheese, wrapped in a refrigerator.
4. Place 1/3 of the cubes of bread in the dish. Cover with half of the sausage and 1/4 cup of the cheese.
5. Pour over the top of 1 cup of the milk mixture.
6. Repeat the layers, yes. Attach the rest of the bread to the end and spill over the last egg and milk mixture.
7. Cover with the salsa with tomato. Cover with plastic wrap and cold overnight.
8. Heat the oven to 350°F in the morning. Uncover the casserole and dust the end with 1/4 cup of shredded cheese.
9. Bake until the strata are golden brown and bubbling and the knife inserted in the middle comes out clean, around 50-60 minutes.

10. Before serving, let rest 10 minutes.

Comments:

A delicious brunch casserole with no fat and no carbohydrates

A real wow factor is applied to the salsa.

ROASTED TOMATILLO SALSA

Ingredients:
- Eight fresh tomatillos, husks removed
- One jalapeno pepper, stem, and seeds removed
- One lemon, grated zest, and juice cooking spray

Direction:
1. Oven to 350°F preheat.
2. On a small baking sheet, put the tomatillos and the jalapeno. Cooking spray. Roast for 20-25 minutes or smooth and golden tomatillos.
3. Move the tomatillos and jalapeno to the food processor.
4. Add citrus fruits and juice—mixing pulse.
5. Cool when ready to use. Cool.

EGGS TUDOR

Ingredients:
- Two Tbs unsalted butter, divided eight jumbo black olives chopped
- Two Tbs flour
- Eight eggs
- One c half and half ¼ c 1% milk dash of salt
- One c turkey ham, slivered
- ¼ tsp white pepper, divided
- ¾ c grated Swiss cheese, divided

- 1/8 tsp nutmeg two cherry tomatoes, halved

Directions:
1. Preheat the broiler.
2. Cold and blend into the flour for one tablespoon of butter, steadily stirring for Half and a Half. Add 1/2 of the pepper and nutmeg, add a splash of salt, and steam until the sauce boils and thickens. Incorporate 1/2 cup of Swiss cheese and diced olives. Stir until the cheese melts over a low fire.
3. Whisk together the eggs and milk and apply the remaining pepper to the eggs. The remaining tablespoon of butter is melted, and the egg mixture is added. Cook until the eggs are set, stirring regularly from the pan's bottom, over low heat.
4. Arrange turkey ham on a 9'x13' bottom baking tray. Cover the sauce with eight teaspoons.
5. Spread on top the leftover sauce, then spread the remainder of the cheese. Layer the eggs on top.
6. Place under the broiler and cook until finely browned at the tip. Garnish with half a cherry tomato each.

Comments:
A favorite for family holidays. This one is a splurge, so be sure to offset the remainder of the day with carbohydrates and calories!

SPINACH SALAD

Ingredients:
- Dressing Salad
- Two Tbs olive oil
- Eight c fresh spinach
- Two Tbs white wine vinegar
- ¼ c diced red onion
- Two Tbs apple cider vinegar
- 1/3 c dried cranberries
- One tsp dry mustard

- Half c candied pecans
- One tsp dry garlic powder
- Half medium apple, cubed
- ¼ tsp salt
- 1/8 tsp black pepper

Directions:
1. Bring the dressing ingredients together in a small pan. Cover and shake thoroughly.
2. Combine the ingredients for the salad in a large tub. Pour over the dressing and toss all to blend.

Comments:
It has been enjoyed by everyone who has tried this salad. In the seasoning, olive oil gives you some heart-healthy fat that you can use every day in your diet. Most people consume just about ten different meals, so you don't even have to try many fresh ideas to improve your eating. One fresh meal takes up 10% of your dinners! It's what you can do!

KALE, LENTIL, & CHICKEN SALAD WITH MAPLE VINAIGRETTE

Ingredients:
- Vinaigrette Salad
- Four Tbs olive oil
- Twelve c kale, sliced in thin
- One Tbs pure maple syrup ribbons
- One Tbs grainy mustard
- Half c raw lentils
- Two tsp red wine vinegar
- Two boneless, skinless chicken breasts
- Two oz reduced-fat feta cheese, crumbled ground black pepper

Directions:

1. Broil or simmer until cooked through, chicken breasts; cool and dice or shred
2. Cook the lentils for about 10-15 minutes in a boiling water pot soft, but not mushy. Drain.
3. Toast almonds until softly golden in the oven or sauté pan-don't overdo them!!
4. In a small pot, put the vinaigrette ingredients, cover, and shake to blend (or whisk together in a small bowl).
5. With the vinaigrette, toss the kale and split equally between 4 bowls. Place on top of chicken, lens, feta, and almonds. Cover the season with black pepper.

Comments:

Chat about greens with leaves!! For autumn, this is a beautiful salad.

QUINOA SALAD WITH RICE & BLACK BEANS

Serves: 6

Ingredients:

- Half c quinoa rinsed well in a sieve 14
- Half oz can vegetable broth
- One and a half tsp ground cumin, divided ½ c long-grain brown rice Fifteen oz can black beans, drained and rinsed well two thin green onions, sliced
- One medium red bell pepper, diced
- Two plum tomatoes, diced
- Half c frozen corn kernels
- ¼ c cilantro
- ¼ c fresh lime juice
- Two Tbs olive oil
- ¼ tsp salt freshly ground
- black pepper, to taste

- 1/8 tsp cayenne pepper.

Directions:
1. Combine the quinoa, 1 cup of the broth, and half a teaspoon of the cumin in a shallow saucepan. Put to a boil, cover, reduce to medium-low heat and simmer for 15-20 minutes before the broth is completely absorbed.
2. To make 1 cup, combine the remaining broth and enough water. Place the rice and a half teaspoon of cumin in a second small saucepan; bring to a boil. Cover and boil for about 15-20 minutes before the liquid is absorbed.
3. In a large tub, add the quinoa and rice together. Add the black beans, bell pepper, green onions, tomatoes, corn, and cilantro.
4. Place in a small container the lime juice, olive oil, the remaining half a teaspoon of cumin, salt, black pepper, and cayenne. Cover and shake to blend. Pour over the salad and mix well. Tips / Comments: The high protein grain quinoa (keen-wa) is used in this recipe with beans to have fiber and magnesium. It can digest more efficiently and blunt the sudden increase of blood sugar because of the fiber. It's a healthy lunch substitute for a burger. A healthy lunch is made by adding a bit of string cheese and a little piece of fruit.

Comments:
This recipe uses quinoa (keen-wa), a high protein grain, with beans that have fiber and magnesium. It can digest more efficiently and blunt the sudden increase of blood sugar because of the fiber. It's a healthy lunch substitute for a burger. A healthy lunch is made by adding a bit of string cheese and a little piece of fruit.

ITALIAN SALAD

Ingredients:
- Half c salad vinegar
- Half c salad oil
- Half tsp salt

- ¼ tsp oregano
- Half tsp garlic powder 1 serving size packet of Truvia or another sweetener
- Two Tbs water three cucumbers, cut into large chunks three tomatoes, cut into large chunks three stalks celery, cut into large chunks.
- One green pepper, cut into large chunks
- One onion, cut into large chunks * other vegetables such as zucchini, cauliflower, etc., work well.

Directions:

1. Marinate the vegetables with dressing for up to 2 hours.
2. Don't drain them.
3. serve.

LENTILS, MINT & FETA FOR 2

Serves: 2

Ingredient:

- One c lentils
- Three and a Half c water
- Half Tbs olive oil
- Half c crumbled feta cheese
- Half c handful of fresh mint

Directions:

1. Water, simmer.
2. Lower the heat and add lentils. Boil until the lentils are tender, or around half an hour.
3. Drain and toss the lentils with olive oil.
4. Chop the mint coarsely.
5. Mix the feta and minced mint.
6. Relax, enjoy.

Comments:

Because it's simple, easy, tasty, and cheap, I like this recipe. I like lentils, and they happen to be low in sugar, low in cholesterol, and low in sodium, too.

Both lentils and mint are extremely rich in iron, which can be beneficial for iron deficiency anemia patients. I'd recommend taking soda and other overly processed yet nutritionally hollow items out of your diet gradually start hunting for raw foods that you can prepare yourself easily even though you're not the most qualified chef in the world.

In the long run, almost everything you assemble from essential and balanced ingredients can prove to be a better option than typically heavily refined and packaged foods that are so predominant in most of our everyday lives.

The fantastic thing about eating healthier is that certain healthy foods for people with diabetes are suitable for most people. It's a remarkable one who is not coping with his diet and makes healthy decisions. Even most doctors (including myself) fail, I suppose. Find a friend, girlfriend, or family who will support you and do things together in a balanced life. A crucial aspect of being good with diabetes is a responsibility to others,

Suppose it's trying to shed weight or take careful care of the carbohydrates. Just take heart! By reading this cookbook and trying to make healthier decisions, you are doing the right thing!

ROASTED CAULIFLOWER, CHICKPEAS & OLIVES

Serves: 6

Ingredients:
- Five c cauliflower florets (about 1 lb)
- Twenty four green olives pitted and sliced four cloves garlic; minced one can garbanzo beans, drained (15 oz)
- Three Tbs olive oil
- Half tsp crushed red pepper
- ¼ tsp chopped fresh parsley

Directions:
1. Preheat the furnace to 450° F.
2. In a shallow roasting pan, mix the first four ingredients, drizzle with olive oil and sprinkle with salt and red pepper. Mix well and cook for 20 minutes or until the cauliflower has browned a little, stirring for 10 minutes.
3. Parsley top.

Comments:
Try using half almond flour and half standard flour when baking cakes and muffins. It reduces carbohydrates and tastes very good.

GRILLED CHILES RELLENOS

Ingredients:
- Six poblano chiles
- Fifteen oz kidney beans rinsed and drained
- Eight oz Monterey Jack cheese grated
- ¼ c raisins
- ¼ c salsa
- Two tsp chili powder

Directions:
1. Lengthwise, cut a slit in each chili, and gently scoop out the seeds and ribs. Mix the beans, cheese, raisins, salsa, and chili powder in a medium dish.
2. Stuff the filler with the peppers
3. Put on a baking sheet, either grill on a barbecue or roast for about 20 minutes in the oven at 350°F. When the pepper is warm, and the cheese is melting, they are finished. Pepper from grilling can look slightly charred.

Comments:

My family loves this recipe because it is delicious, but I love it because it is versatile and straightforward. Experiment with fillings that are different. At Farmer's markets, we find numerous sweet and spicy peppers and have served well. We also buy extra frozen peppers because we've got them all year long.

BAKED LEEK & SWEET POTATO GRATIN

Serves: 8

Ingredients:

- Three medium leeks, white and light green parts only chopped (about 6 cups)
- One and a Half Tbs olive oil, divided three cloves garlic, minced
- Three Tbs chopped fresh rosemary, separated Two lbs medium sweet potatoes, peeled and cut into 1/8-inch slices
- 1/3 c low-sodium vegetable broth
- Three Tbs Italian seasoned dry bread crumbs
- Two Tbs Romano cheese (optional) cooking spray

Directions:

1. Preheat the oven to 450°F. Cover 10' of the round baking dish with spray for cooking
2. Take a medium-high heat tablespoon of oil in a season. Add leeks, garlic, and 1 1/2 tablespoons of rosemary; sauté for 8 minutes. If necessary, season with a pinch of salt and pepper.
3. Place over the bottom of the prepared baking dish one-third of the sweet potato slices, slightly overlapping. Place on the Top Half of the leek mixture. Arrange over leeks another 1/3 of the sweet potato slices. Top with remaining leeks and then cover with remaining sweet potato slices. Drizzle broth over the plate, cover with foil and bake for 35 minutes.
4. In a small cup, whisk together bread crumbs, remaining olive oil, remaining rosemary, and Romano cheese, if needed. Remove

foil from the gratin and scatter over the top with breadcrumb mixture. Bake for 15 more minutes uncovered. Before eating, let cool, cut into wedges, and enjoy.

APPLE-GLAZED BABY CARROTS

Ingredients:
- Three c baby carrots
- One Tbs lemon juice
- One Tbs low-calorie margarine
- Three Tbs apple juice concentrate
- 2/3 c low-sodium chicken broth
- One tsp cinnamon
- Two tsp cornstarch or arrowroot powder 1 tsp water

Directions:
1. Steam the carrots for about 3 minutes over 2 inches of boiling water, sealed.
2. Sprinkle the juice with the lemon.
3. In a medium bath, melt the margarine at low heat
4. Connect the condensed apple juice and boil until it melts.
5. Attach the cinnamon and broth and carry to a boil. 6. Combine the cornstarch Or powder arrowroot with water. Lower the flame, apply it to the pan, and cook until it thickens. To coat, add the carrots and toss well.

ROASTED CARROTS WITH SHALLOTS & SAGE

Serves: 2

Ingredients:
- ¾ c baby carrots
- Two large shallots halved lengthwise
- One Tbs balsamic vinegar

- One tsp olive oil
- One Tbs hacked the new smart garlic pinch the pinch with salt and black peppers

Directions:

1. Preheat the oven to 400 degrees F.
2. In an 8" or 9" oven-safe skillet, toss the carrots and shallots with the vinegar and oil.
3. When cooking, roast for 25 to 30 minutes or until the vegetables are tender and deeply browned, turning once.
4. Place in a small cup, put it, and toss it with the last four ingredients.

Comments:

Only right for two persons.

MASHED CAULIFLOWER POTATOES

Serves: 4

Ingredients:

- One medium red potato (about 8 ounces) cut into 1-inch chunks 8 oz cauliflower florets
- ¼ c onion chopped
- One tsp dried parsley
- ¼ tsp garlic powder
- Two Tbs margarine pepper to taste

Directions:

1. In a medium saucepan, mix the potato, cauliflower, onion, parsley, and garlic powder with enough water to barely coat them. Take a simmer, then reduce the heat and cook.
2. Cook for about 12 minutes, until the vegetables are soft. Drain thoroughly.
3. Mash with a masher of potatoes. Incorporate margarine and mash until smooth. To taste, season with pepper.

Comments:

For an added spice, consider adding a little Parmesan or chopped garlic.

GARLIC MUSHROOMS

Serves: 12

Ingredients:

- Two lb button mushrooms wiped clean and halved if large
- ¼ c olive oil
- Half c chopped kalamata olives
- Two Tbs balsamic vinegar
- One tsp dried thyme one clove garlic, minced

Directions:

1. To 450 degrees F preheat the oven. On a non-stick baking sheet with a rim, put the mushrooms and toss with the olive oil. Lightly dust with pepper and salt.
2. Roast for 15 minutes on a baking dish. Stir and roast for an extra 10 minutes or until brown and crisp.
3. Mix the remainder, then feed at room temperature or elevated temperature.

Comments:

For brunch or dinner, this is a perfect side dish. Usually, I omit olives.

DECADENT BRUSSELS SPROUTS

Serve: 4

Ingredients:

- Twenty brussels sprouts, trimmed and cut in Half
- One c half and half ½ lemon, juiced pepper to taste

Directions:

1. Place the Brussels on the side and cut it to medium heat up to bubble until the sprinkling is half in a 10" saute pan.
2. Lower heat to reduced and simmer until sprouts are dull tender for around 20 minutes.
3. Stir in the top and apply freshly ground pepper to extract from the sun.

Comments:

Even my picky eater likes those, amazingly simple and happy.

SWEET POTATO SPEARS

Serves: 4

Ingredients:

- One and a half lbs of peeled and cut into lengthwise spears sweet potatoes
- One tbs of olive oil
- Half tsp of salt
- 1/4 tsp of dried thyme
- 1/4 tsp of pepper
- 1/8 tsp of nutmeg

Directions

1. Insert all the ingredients in a container, mix, and coat the potato slices.
2. Arrange on a baking sheet sprayed with a cooking spray or lined with parchment in a single layer. Put it on the lower shelf of the oven and bake at 450°F for 25 minutes or until soft, stirring once.

CURRIED LENTILS & CAULIFLOWER

Ingredients:

- One cup dry lentils
- One bay leaf
- Two cups of water
- Two tsp of olive oil
- One chopped onion
- One clove of garlic minced
- One tsp of salt
- One tsp of ground coriander
- One tsp of ground cumin
- One tsp of turmeric
- 1/4 tsp of cinnamon
- One tiny flower head cut in flowerets.
- One and a half cup of tomato sauce
- One tsp of freshly grated ginger root optional garnish: 1/2 cup of roasted cashews,
- Half cup of plain yogurt

Directions

1. Clean and drain the lentils. Place in a pot with bay leaf and water and bring to a boil. Lower heat, cover, and boil for 25-30 minutes until the lentils are tender. 2. Heat the oil in a big pot. Add the onion, garlic, and salt; sauté until the onion has softened. .Add coriander, cumin.
2. Turmeric, cinnamon. Then add cauliflower, tomato sauce, ginger, and 3/4 cup of water, stir well.
3. Cook and cover until the cauliflower is tender, about 15 more minutes. Stir the cooked lentils in the cauliflower mixture and remove the bay leaf. Top with garnishes if you want to.

CHICKEN & WHITE BEAN SOUP

Ingredients:

- Twelve oz boneless, skinless chicken breasts
- Two tsp Smart Balance Omega Oil
- Two leeks washed and cut into ¼" rounds (white and light green part)
- One Tbs chopped fresh sage (or ¼ tsp dried sage)
- Two Tbs sodium-free chicken bouillon
- Two c water one can (15 ½ oz) no-salt-added cannellini (white kidney) beans, rinsed

Directions:

1. Until cooked, boil the chicken breasts: set aside until cool. If the chicken is fresh, shred it.
2. In a soup pot or a large Netherlands oven, heat oil over medium-high heat. Stir leeks and frequently cook for about 3 minutes until soft.
3. Remove the sage and carry on cooking for about 30 seconds until aromatic.
4. Stir in the water and the bouillon. Increase the heat, cover it, and bring it to a boil.
5. Add chicken and beans; cook, occasionally stirring, until hot, about 5 minutes. Serve it warm.

Comments:

Quick and simple-Modify the herbs you add if you want a different flavor. The soup can all be delicious with basil, garlic, cilantro, estragon, or oregano! Right from the brisk fall of the wall.

TACO SOUP

Serves: 4

Ingredients:
- Sixteen oz ground turkey
- One large onion chopped
- Two to three ribs celery chopped
- Two tsp low sodium Old El Paso taco seasoning (2)
- Sixteen oz cans tomatoes no salt added
- One to two Tbs cider vinegar
- Thirty-two oz of low sodium chicken broth rinsed with soft sodium chili beans.
- One c frozen corn garnishes sour cream, limes, and cilantro sprigs

Directions:
1. In a big soup pot, brown turkey. Celery, onion, and cook for about eight more minutes more.
2. Add taco, tomatoes, vinegar, and broth, and cook for approximately 20 minutes. Add beans and maize. Cook 15 minutes more. Cook.
3. In bowls, put on a bag of cilantro and sour cream. For squeezing over the top, serve with limes.

Comments:
It is even better the second day, like with most soup recipes!

EGG, LEMON & RICE SOUP (AVGOLEMONO SOUPA)

Serves: 8

Ingredients:
- Two qts low sodium chicken broth
- Half c long-grain brown rice
- Four large eggs
- 2/3 c freshly squeezed lemon juice salt and pepper

Directions:

1. Bring broth and rice to a boil in a medium bowl over high heat. Decrease heat, cover, and cook until rice is soft (per rice package instructions). Put in a pinch of salt and pepper, heat away.
2. In a bowl, mix the eggs with the citrus fruit and 1/4 taste of water. In a cup of hot broth, gradually whisk. Then mix the egg in broth and rice slowly.

    Stir in low heat for only 1-3 minutes until hot. You may not boil or curdle soup.
3. Put in and serve in bowls.

Comments:

It is a suitable food starter - tropical flavor carbs. Here's a tip, plan, and balance your food to prevent spikes of glucose.

BEEF BARLEY SOUP

Serves: 8

Ingredients:

- Two lb beef stew meat, cut into 1" cubes
- One Tbs olive oil
- One large or two small leeks, root and dark green ends cut off, and leek sliced lengthwise, rinsed thoroughly, and sliced thinly
- Two c chopped carrot
- Four cloves garlic minced
- Six c water
- One and a half tsp salt
- One tsp dried thyme
- Half tsp ground black pepper
- Four bay leaves
- 28 oz low-sodium beef broth
- One c pearl barley

Directions:

1. Over medium heat, heat a big Dutch oven with oil. Add 5 minutes of half the beef and cook, brown everywhere. Repeat the other half of the beef in a bowl.
2. Stir and reduce the heat if needed to prevent too much browning; add leek, carrot, and garlic to your pan. Add water, the next five ingredients (to brown), and beef to the pan if the vegetables are lightly browned.
3. Boil, heat, cover, and cook for 1 hour. Bring to boil. Add the barley or until the beef and barley are tender. Cook another thirty to 40 minutes. Before serving, throw out the bay leaves.

CHICKEN & VEGETABLE SOUP

Serves: 4

Ingredients:

- Two Tbs olive oil
- One lb chicken tenders, cut into bite-size pieces
- Two small zucchinis, diced small
- Two shallots or half a red onion, diced small
- Three plum tomatoes, chopped
- One tsp Italian herb blend
- Twenty-eight oz low-sodium chicken broth
- Half c white wine (or use a little more chicken broth) 4 Tbs small pasta shape (orzo, for example)
- Three c baby spinach (or larger leaves, chopped roughly), rinsed.

Directions:

1. Heat oil over medium heat in large bowls.
2. Stir in the chicken and cook until browned, occasionally stirring about three to four minutes. Take a bowl and transfer it.
3. In a saucepan, often melt until the vegetables are slightly softened; add the courgettes, shallot or red onion, tomatoes, and herb blend.

4. Bring a boil to the soup, add wine, broth, and pasta, and stir sometimes. Check the cooking time package to reduce heat to a stir and cook till the pasta is tender.
5. Cook until all is thoroughly heated and chicken is fully cooked for a further 4-5 minutes. Add chicken and spinach.

Comments:

The right way to eat your food

CURRY PUMPKIN SOUP

Serves: 6

Ingredients:

- One large onion
- One Tbs butter
- One c chopped carrots
- Six c low sodium chicken broth
- Three and a half c canned pumpkin
- Half c half and half ½ c white wine
- Two tsp brown sugar
- One Tbs curry powder (add more if you prefer a more robust flavor)

Directions:

1. Sprinkle onion in butter until nice (approximately 15 minutes at medium-high) and caramelize.
2. Add carrots and cook for another ten minutes
3. Put a cup of the broth into the pot's bottom to deglaze (this should scrape into the soup with the fatty brown bits).
4. Then add the rest of the broth and the rest, except the half and half ingredients. Take a kick.
5. Reduce to decreases and cook for 30 minutes. Remove half and half. Remove. Curry and adjust the pepper to your taste. Ladle in and enjoy the large bowls.

Comments:

Great, but to make it more significant, you can add a little chicken or white beans. On one side, there is a whole grain roll to tumble. Easy and creative cooking is healthy. In our cuisine, it is essential to spend more time.

TURKEY CHILI

Serves: 4

Ingredients:
- Two c chopped cooked turkey
- One clove garlic, minced
- One medium onion, chopped
- One green pepper, diced
- One can (17 oz) can red kidney beans
- One can (6 oz) can tomato paste
- One can (28 oz) can tomatoes
- One bay leaf
- One Tbs chili powder, more if you like a little more heat
- Half tsp cumin seeds

Directions:
1. In a large pot of soup, combine turkey, garlic, onion, and green pepper. Sprinkle until soft vegetables. Stir in and cover with other ingredients.
2. Simmer 30-60 minutes over low heat or until flavors mix.

Comments:

Fall is always a good chili time. I get out my crockpot and start chili if there's a brisk feeling of falling in the air. "No secrets to success. Yum!

ITALIAN CHICKEN WITH CHICKPEAS

Serves: 4

Ingredients:
- One and a half tsp minced garlic
- One lb chicken tenders
- ¼ tsp salt
- ¼ tsp black pepper
- One Tbs olive oil
- One c green pepper strips
- Fifteen and a half oz can chickpeas
- Fourteen and a half oz can diced tomatoes with basil and oregano

Directions:
1. Pour salt and pepper over the chicken—heat oil on medium warmth in a vast, non-stick pot. Fill in the pan with chicken and cook on each side for around 2 minutes, until browned. Add onion and pepper and sprinkle for 4 minutes. Shrink heat to medium.
2. Cover and cook for 8 minutes or until thoroughly heated; add garlic, chickpeas, and tomatoes.

Comments:
Significant to be accompanied by a whole grain!

CHICKEN TORTILLAS

Makes: 12

Ingredients:
- ¼ c lime juice
- One-two cloves garlic minced
- One tsp chili powder

- Half tsp ground cumin
- Three lbs boneless skinless chicken breasts cut into ¼ inch strips
- One large onion, sliced
- One green bell pepper, sliced
- One red bell pepper, sliced
- Twelve whole wheat 8" tortillas
- One c salsa ½ c fat-free sour cream
- Half c low fat shredded cheese

Directions:

1. Combine the initial four ingredients in a large bowl. Stir in chicken slices until well coated with chicken. Fifteen minutes marinate.
2. Cook in the grill or stovetop chicken in a pan until they are not pink anymore. Add onions and peppers to cook 5 minutes more.
3. Split the mix into tortillas evenly. Hold the salsa, savory cream, and shredded cheese on top.
4. Serve and roll-up.

SALSA TURKEY MEATLOAF

Serves: 6

Ingredients:

- One lb ground turkey
- One egg
- Half c fine dry bread crumbs
- One finely diced onion
- One garlic clove, minced
- ¾ c salsa, divided

Directions:

1. To 400 °F, preheat the oven.
2. Coat with cooking spray a 9 "x5" loaf pot.

3. Put turkey, egg, breadcrumbs, garlic, and 1/2 cup of salsa in a large saucepan. Mix carefully. 3.
4. In the pan and spread the turkey mixture evenly.
5. Bake for 50-60 minutes, add the remaining salsa, and bake.

BARBEQUE PULLED CHICKEN

Serves: 8

Ingredients:

- Eight oz can low-sodium tomato sauce
- Three Tbs cider vinegar
- Two Tbs honey
- One Tbs sweet OR smoked paprika
- One Tbs tomato paste
- One Tbs Worcestershire sauce
- Two tsp dry mustard
- One tsp ground dried chipotle chile
- Half tsp salt
- Two and a half lbs boneless, skinless chicken thighs, trimmed of fat
- One small onion, minced
- One clove garlic, minced

Directions:

1. Stir tomato sauce, chilies, vinegar, sweetheart, paprika, tomato paste, Worcestershire, mustard, chipotle, and salt to 6 square meters. Slow to smooth, cooker slowly. Stir in a combination of chicken, onion, and garlic.
2. On the cooker, put the lid and cook for 5 hours on LOW.
3. Pull the chicken over to the board with forks and remove the chicken. Turn the chicken back into the sauce, stir, and serve well!

CILANTRO CITRUS CHICKEN

Serves: 4

Ingredients:

- ¼ c onion, chopped
- One Tbs fresh cilantro leaves
- One Tbs fresh parsley leaves
- One Tbs fresh orange juice
- One Tbs fresh lime juice
- Two cloves garlic 4 (4 oz each) chicken breast halves 2/3 tsp salt substitute
- 1/3 tsp ground cumin
- Half tsp ground pepper cooking spray

Directions:

1. Combine in a food mill or blender or blender until the first seven ingredients are smooth. In a ziplock bag, place the chicken and half the grass mix. Refrigerate for 1 hour, seal and marinate, and occasionally turn the bag. Remove chicken and throw it out of the bag.
2. Let 15 minutes of the chicken stand. Sprinkle the cumin and pepper left with the salt replacement.
3. Sprinkle with a sprayed grill or sauté. Grill or cook in the sauté pot, about 12 minutes on the side until fully cooked.

OVEN-FRIED CHICKEN

Serves: 4

Ingredients:

- Half c buttermilk
- One Tbs Dijon mustard
- Two cloves garlic, minced

- Two and a half -three lb chicken legs, skin removed (use paper towels for a good grip and pull from the thigh down over the drumstick)
- Half c whole wheat flour
- Two Tbs sesame seeds
- One and a half tsp paprika
- One tsp dried thyme
- One tsp baking powder
- ¼ tsp salt freshly ground pepper to taste

Directions:

1. In a small bowl, whisk butter, mustard, and garlic. In the Ziploc bag, put the chicken legs into the buttermilk mix and squeeze the bag tightly, pressing the air gently into the bag. Turn the sac gently from side to side and cover with buttermilk. The chicken a place for a half hour or up to 8 hours in the refrigerator.
2. Baker at 425°F. Preheat. Line the foil of a bakery. Put on the foil a baker and coat with a spray for cooking.
3. In another Ziploc or a plastic bag, combine meal, sésame seeds, paprika, thyme, baked pulp, salt, and pepper. Insert one leg of chicken at a time and shake to cover the portion with the flour mix. Shake off the flour and put on the bakery. Spray additional cooking spray chicken pieces. Remove the remaining buttermilk and meal mixtures.
4. Bake for 40-50 minutes, until golden brown.

Comments / Tips:

Children love the fried chicken alternative!

CHICKEN CASSOULET

Serves: 6

Ingredients:

- Two white beans (15 oz) cans, drained

- 3/4 c panko
- Two Tbs olive oil, divided
- One lb boneless, skinless chicken thighs cut into thirds
- One large onion, chopped
- Four cloves garlic, chopped
- Half tsp dried rosemary
- Half tsp dried thyme
- Half tsp ground black pepper
- Half c dry white wine (or substitute extra chicken broth)
- Half c low-sodium chicken broth
- Half lb low-fat turkey kielbasa, in ½" slices

Directions:

1. Preheat to 375°F. Preheat the oven.
2. In a small bowl, thaw the panko with one tablespoon of olive oil. Give it up.
3. Heat in a nonadhesive skillet the remaining one tablespoon olive oil and add chicken pieces. Prepare till browned, turning as soon as, about 5 minutes complete. Transfer to the bakery, sprayed with spray.
4. In the skillet, add onion and garlic and cook for about 5 minutes until soft. Stir in herbs and pepper, and then cook for 30 seconds. Cook. Stir in wine and cook until halved. Bring the fruit to a boil with broth, beans, and kielbasa. In the baking dish, pour over the chicken and sprinkle the panko over it. Bake until bubbling browned for 20-25 minutes.

CHICKEN LO MEIN WITH PEANUT SAUCE

Serves: 6 (about 2 cups per serving)

Ingredients:

- Cooking spray
- Eight oz wide lo mein noodles
- Fourteen oz can low sodium chicken broth

- Two Tbs reduced-fat peanut butter
- Two Tbs rice wine vinegar
- Two Tbs sweet chili sauce
- Two Tbs low sodium soy sauce
- Two tsp dark sesame oil, divided
- One lb chicken breasts, cut into small pieces
- Two tsp minced garlic
- One tsp grated ginger
- One (Eighteen oz) package fresh stir-fry vegetable medley
- Three Tbs chopped fresh basil
- Two Tbs chopped unsalted, dry roasted peanuts

Directions:

1. Cook lo mein noodles, omitting any added fat or salt according to the package directions.
2. Mix the chicken broth with the following four ingredients in a small bowl; mix well with a whisk.
3. While the noodles are cooked, heat one teaspoon of oil in a large, non-stick, cooking spray pan over medium-high heat. Add the chicken to the pan and sauté for 6 minutes or until done. Remove the pan and set aside.
4. Add one teaspoon of oil remaining in the pot. Sprinkle with garlic and ginger for 30 seconds and sauté. Stir in the mix of vegetables and sprinkle in a pan for 4 minutes or only until tender. Stir in a mixture of peanut butter and bring to a boil—Cook until thickened or 5 minutes. Go back to the pot of the chicken and cook for 2 minutes or until heated thoroughly. Toss well and add noodles.
5. Top each serving with basil and peanuts as desired.

Comment:

It is a recipe that is low-fat, low-sodium, and healthy for everyone. The whole family likes to eat, it's affordable, and it's quick and easy. We prefer to use fresh vegetables instead of frozen vegetables. It's great to have healthy cooking fun for the whole family. Including your spouse, children, and grandchildren can make it more fun!! My son loves to do this.

GRILLED FISH TACOS WITH CHIPOTLE-LIME DRESSING

Serves: 4

Ingredients:
- ¼ c olive oil
- Two Tbs white vinegar
- Two Tbs lime juice
- Two tsp lime zest
- One and a half tsp honey
- Two cloves garlic, minced
- Half tsp cumin
- Half tsp chili powder
- One tsp seafood seasonings, such as Old Bay
- Half tsp ground black pepper
- One tsp hot pepper sauce
- One lb tilapia filets, cut into chunks

Dressing:
- Eight oz light sour cream
- Half c adobo sauce from chipotle peppers
- Two Tbs fresh lime juice
- Two tsp lime zest
- ¼ tsp cumin
- ¼ tsp chili powder
- Half tsp seafood seasoning, such as Old Bay

Toppings:
- One package tortillas
- Three ripe tomatoes, seeded and diced
- One bunch cilantro, chopped
- One small head cabbage, cored and shredded

- Two limes cut in wedges

Directions:

1. Mix the olive oil, the vinegar, the lime juice, the lime zest, the honey, the garlic, the cumin, the chili powder, the seafood seasoning, and the black pepper the hot sauce in a bowl until the marinade is mixed. Place the tilapia and pour the marinade over the fish in a shallow dish—cover and freeze for 6 to 8 hours.
2. To create the dressing, combine the sour cream and adobo sauce in a bowl. Stir in the seasoning with lime juice, lime zest, cumin, chili, and seafood. To taste, season. Cover and keep refrigerated.
3. Preheat a high-heat outdoor grill and lightly grill the oil. "Set the heat to grid 4".
4. Remove the marinade fish, drain off any excess, and discard the marinade. Grill the pieces of fish until a fork is easily flaked, turning once about 9 minutes.
5. Assemble tacos by putting fish pieces with desired quantities of tomatoes, cilantro, and cabbage in the center of tortillas; drizzle with dressing. Roll up tortillas around fillings to serve, and garnish with lime wedges.

Comments:

In this recipe, the marinated fish can also be cooked in the oven. Preheat the 350 ° F oven

Bake for 9 to 11 minutes in a preheated oven until the fish flakes easily with a fork. Assemble tacos according to the instructions. The tilapia can be replaced by mahi-mahi.

Count your blessings and indeed be grateful for your life.

APPLE-GLAZED SALMON

Serves: 2

Ingredients:

- Twelve oz salmon fillet, about 1" thick (fresh or frozen, thawed)

- One tsp juniper berries, dried, crushed
- Two Tbs vermouth
- ¾ tsp fresh thyme, finely snipped
- Half tsp fresh rosemary, finely snipped.
- Two Tbs apple jelly

Directions:

1. Cook the juniper berries in a small dry saucepan over medium-high heat for about 1 minute or toasted. Shake the pan often.
2. Add the vermouth, thyme, and rosemary very carefully. Just bring it to a boil.
3. Combine with apple jelly. Simmer for 1 minute or until the jelly melts. Withdraw from the heat.
4. Rinse the fish with a paper towel and pat it dry. Cut the fish into two chunks.
5. Over high heat, heat a large skillet. Combine the fish, skin-side up—Cook for approximately 2 minutes, or until light brown.
6. Place the fish on the skin side down to a baking plate. Lightly sprinkle the fish with salt and pepper. Spoon the fish over the glaze.
7. Baked in a 400°F oven for 8 to 10 minutes and glazed light brown or until flakes are easy

POACHED WHITEFISH

Serves: 4

Ingredients:

- One lb white fish(halibut, sole, cod) fillet or steaks
- One small sweet onion thinly sliced
- One fresh lemon washed and thinly sliced
- Half to one c non-fat milk dill weed fresh ground pepper

Directions:

1. Preheat the oven to 325 degrees F.

2. Spray with non-stick cooking spray on the bottom of a baking dish. Lay in the plate with the fish. Place the fish with the onion and lemon slices. To cover the fish, add the non-fat milk. Sprinkle with pepper and dill weed.
3. Protect the dish with foil and bake it for about 20 minutes, until the fish flakes easily.
4. Remove from the milk the fish and enjoy (discard the milk).
5. Serve with brown rice and a non-starchy vegetable. Tips / Comments: This is a good source of low-fat protein. Part of a healthy eating plan is to include fish 1-2 times a week. Without frying, this recipe keeps the fish moist.

FARFALLE WITH SALMON, MINT, AND PEAS

Serves: 6

Ingredients:
- One lb farfalle
- One and a half lb skinned salmon, cut in chunks
- ¼ c water
- Two lemons, juice, and zest
- Ten oz package of frozen peas
- ¼ c fresh chopped mint
- Two Tbs butter

Directions:
1. Cook the pasta on the package as directed.
2. Put the salmon in a large skillet and season with salt and pepper. Incorporate water, lemon juice, and zest. Simmer, cover, and cook for 10 minutes. Add the peas, cover them, and cook for 6-8 more minutes. Add the butter and mint to the drained pasta. Toss gently with extra chopped mint and serve.

Comments:
Very good.

GRILLED SALMON STEAKS WITH TARRAGON SAUCE

Serves: 4

Ingredients

- Four salmon steaks, about 1" thick
- Three Tbs lemon juice
- Two shallots, minced
- Two Tbs chopped fresh tarragon or (2 tsp dried)
- One c plain non-fat yogurt
- One medium plum tomato, seeded and minced
- One Tbs minced flat-leaf parsley

Directions:

1. Preheat the broiler, or begin grilling.
2. Use lemon juice to brush both sides of the salmon: broil or grill.
3. Combine the shallots, tarragon, yogurt, tomato, and parsley while the salmon cooks.
4. Arrange the salmon and top with the sauce on the plates.

Comments:

A big favorite from the Northwest, topped with a guilt-free, tasty garnish

Lightning Source UK Ltd.
Milton Keynes UK
UKHW020642110221
378620UK00014B/955